The Missing Link between the Mind, the Body, and the Needle

Dr. Michelle Han, DAOM

Dr Michelle Han, DAOM.

Dedication

To my Han family—the lineage I carry in my breath, my bones, and the way I hold stories that were never written down.

To the ones who came before me, who worked with the body before it was called medicine, who held grief in silence, and passed down wisdom in gesture, not words.

To the land that raised me, and the language that shaped me even in its absence.

To my father, whose stillness taught me how to listen.

To the women in my bloodline who felt everything and were told to feel nothing.

To the patients who trusted me before I had the words for what I was holding.

To the girl who was forced to read the room to survive.

To the woman who alchemized survival into power.

To the Witch Doctor who came home through the body.

This book is the map I didn't inherit, but chose to draw anyway.

The missing link I became by remembering.

The truth I had to live in order to write.

TABLE OF CONTENTS

Introduction The New Paradigm of Healing

"I was doing all the 'right' things. Journaling, meditating, going to therapy, burning the sage, and doing the inner child work. But my body... my body was still flinching like I hadn't healed a thing."

This book was not born from theory.

It was born from the tremor in my nervous system that therapy couldn't soothe.

It was born from the clients who spoke their trauma beautifully — but still couldn't sleep, breathe, or feel safe in their own skin.

It was born from the deep grief in my gut that acupuncture released — even though I had no words for it at the time.

I didn't always know I was here to create a new modality.

In fact, I spent years trying to fit into someone else's method, someone else's "proven system." I thought I needed to stay clinical enough to be credible and spiritual enough to be seen as "evolved." I contorted myself between two worlds.

But the truth is:

I am a witch doctor in a white coat, a neuroscience geek with spirit guides, a licensed practitioner with a priestess heart.

And I know I'm not alone.

I've spent over a decade in the worlds of psychology, energy medicine, and trauma healing. I've sat in front of clients who could articulate their trauma with surgical precision... but still found themselves looping in the same patterns, the same freeze states, the same burnouts.

Let me take you into a room you've likely been in before.

A therapy office. A softly lit space. You're asked how you feel. You answer. You excavate memory. You name the patterns. You leave with insight, sometimes relief, sometimes exhaustion.

But your body still hurts.

Or perhaps it's the treatment table. You lie back. Needles are placed. Your practitioner reads your tongue, your pulse, your Qi. You feel better. Your digestion improves. Your migraines soften. But there's a grief that doesn't budge. An anxiety that continues whispering.

Both are trying to help you. But neither speaks the other's language.

This is the broken bridge I found myself standing on for years. A chasm between two powerful worlds:

- The psychological and the somatic.
- The mind and the meridians.
- The narrative and the nervous system.

Western psychology taught us to name the trauma, tell the story, and sit with the discomfort. Eastern medicine taught us to move the energy, release the heat, and regulate the channels.

But what about the trauma stored in the heat? What about the heartbreak held in the liver? What about the grief that isn't a thought, but a pattern in the breath?

Modern wellness has tried to merge these traditions. We see terms like "trauma-informed acupuncture" or "mind-body healing". But most of what is offered is done so through metaphor, not method. They talk about the mind-body connection but offer no bridge.

I wanted the bridge. I needed it. My patients needed it.

And I began to ask a simple, revolutionary question:

What if the point prescription also held an emotional code?

What if the healing model itself is incomplete?

I began to watch more closely. To ask softer questions. To track not just pulse quality, but the breath changing with each insertion.

And slowly, the bridge began to rebuild itself. Not from textbooks, but from tears. From sighs. From trembles. From the way a patient would suddenly remember a moment from childhood, right as the heart meridian opened.

This chapter is the map of that search. The moments where acupuncture failed to meet the emotion. The sessions where therapy failed to reach the body. The cracks I walked until I began to understand:

You cannot talk the body into safety.

You cannot needle the soul without listening.

And so, Psychology Acupuncture was born: a synthesis of soul work, somatic healing, archetypal remembrance, and energetic precision. This is a new modality. A bridge between East and West, science and spirit, analysis and ritual. A remembrance of healing as it was always meant to be: embodied, mythic, intuitive, and true. This book is for the healers who have felt split. For the clinicians who sense there is more. For the witches hiding in white coats and the mystics dressed in modern skin. For you, who feels the missing link. It is a map back to yourself.

You do not need to become anything other than what you already are. You need only remember.

If you're reading this, something inside you remembers too.

Something is whispering:

There's more.

There's a missing link.

You are carrying it.

What This Book Will Do

In these pages, I will take you into the core of what I call Psychology Acupuncture — a method that bridges:

- Mental health science with energetic intelligence
- Cognitive insight with somatic release
- Client empowerment with soul remembrance

You'll read case stories that defy logic but feel deeply true.

You'll understand how trauma gets stored in the meridians, not just the memories.

You'll witness how a single point on the body can collapse a karmic loop, dissolve grief, or awaken long silenced voice.

A Note to the Reader

This is not just a book.

It's a portal.

Some chapters will feel like a remembering.

Others may stir a sacred discomfort — a signal that a truth is rising.

You may not agree with every word, and that's okay. I'm not here to convince. I'm here to mirror back the wisdom already encoded within you — the part that knows healing can be both clinical and mystical, structured and sacred.

This book is for the seekers who've outgrown systems. Psychology acupuncture is a term used to describe an acupuncture-based framework for understanding the somatic and physiological correlates of psychological experience. It does not refer to the practice of psychology or psychotherapy, which requires separate licensure.

This book is for the healers who are ready to reclaim the medicine they ARE, not just the modalities they learned.

It's for the part of you that has always whispered:

There's something missing… and maybe I'm the one who came to bring it back.

Welcome to the bridge.

Let's walk it together.

Let us begin where all true healing does: at the point where pain becomes purpose.

Part I

The Fragmented Healing Paradigm

Chapter 1
The Talk Therapy Ceiling

We are a culture obsessed with fragmentation. The mind is separated from the body. The body is separated from the soul. And healing is often reduced to protocols, metrics, or diagnoses that slice the self into clinical categories. We've inherited a split system that treats mental health like a software glitch and physical health like a hardware failure.

But healing was never meant to be this dismembered. Healing, in its original form, is remembrance. A return. A reunion of the holy trinity within us: mind, body, and spirit.

In the West, psychology has reigned as the lens through which we understand behavior, emotion, and identity. It gives language to trauma, tools for transformation, and frameworks for the psyche. But it often stops at the neck. The body becomes a symptom-holder rather than a partner in the healing process.

Meanwhile, in Eastern medicine, acupuncture speaks fluently to the body's energy systems. It maps pain to pathways, emotions to organs, and sees illness as a reflection of imbalance. Yet even this, in modern practice, is often confined to physical relief: back pain, insomnia, digestion, stress. What of destiny? What of the unseen grief curled in the womb? What of the soul's ache to be remembered?

What if we stopped asking: "What is the diagnosis?" and instead asked: "What is the soul trying to say through the symptom?"

"The mind can understand the trauma, but the body still flinches."

I've met hundreds of people who could explain their trauma with brilliance.

They could name their attachment style, describe their coping mechanisms, recite their therapist's language about boundaries and nervous system states.

But they were still waking up with panic attacks.

Still freezing when someone they loved got too close.

Still playing out abandonment loops they already understood.

And I began to wonder:

If understanding was enough, why weren't we healed yet?

Talk Therapy Was a Revolution — But Not a Completion

Let's name this with care: therapy saves lives.

It has provided language where there was once only silence.

It has given many of us the first space to be truly heard.

But as a practitioner, and as a client myself, I began to see the pattern:

- Years of therapy, yet still stuck in patterns
- Emotional breakthroughs with no nervous system follow-through

- Clients "performing insight" while their bodies screamed in suppression

We were treating trauma like a puzzle. But trauma is not intellectual. It is sensory. Somatic. Cyclical. And it doesn't live in your thoughts – it lives in your tissues.

The Loop: Understanding without Embodiment

Here's how the loop often plays out:

1. You name the pattern: abandonment, perfectionism, people-pleasing
2. You trace it to childhood or early relational wounds
3. You feel temporarily seen or relieved
4. But nothing really changes

Why?

Because talking about the wound is not the same as truly healing the wound.

Because even as the brain processes, the body is still bracing for the same danger it knew before you had the words.

We call this "false clarity" – when you know what's wrong, but can't shift it. And it becomes its own trap: a prison made of language.

Healing Is Not Just Insight – It's Safety

Healing doesn't ask: "Do you understand what happened?"

It asks:

- "Can you feel safe while it's happening?"
- "Can your body stay present without dissociating?"

- "Can your breath stay open while you remember?"

Talk therapy often gives us context.

But context without safety is still dysregulation.

I've seen clients cry for the first time only after a single needle was placed at Pericardium 8.

Not because they remembered anything new – but because the energetic armor finally released.

Because their body felt safe enough to feel.

Where Talk Therapy Meets Its Edge

Here's what the traditional therapy room can struggle to reach:

- Pre-verbal trauma – experiences that happened before you had language
- Somatic memory – stored in fascia, muscles, meridians, not memory
- Energetic residue – relational cords, karmic loops, ancestral grief
- Nervous system re-patterning – requires more than insight; it requires re-experiencing in safety

This is where acupuncture – especially when combined with psychological attunement – becomes profound. The needle speaks directly to the part of you that never had words.

Case Example: The Woman Who Couldn't Cry

Let me tell you about Hana.

She had been in therapy for six years.

She was articulate, insightful, and completely disconnected from her body.

She said, "I can tell you everything about my trauma. I just can't feel it."

I placed three needles:

- Pericardium 6 – to soothe the Heart and Shen
- Liver 3 – to release suppressed rage
- Kidney 1 – to root her into the Earth

Within minutes, her chest began to shake.

She sobbed — not from memory, but from release.

Her body, for the first time in years, remembered it was safe enough to weep.

Her breakthrough didn't come from a question.

It came from energetic permission.

Why We Intellectualize Pain

There's a reason we stay in our heads:

- The mind is where we first gained control
- Insight gives us a sense of safety
- Understanding makes us feel productive

But healing is not productivity.

And the need to understand everything is often a trauma response in disguise.

When we intellectualize pain, we protect ourselves from feeling it.

But what is un-felt becomes un-integrated.

And what is un-integrated… repeats.

What the Body Needs

The body doesn't need insight.

It needs:

- Safety
- Slowness
- Sensory integration
- Energetic coherence

And this is where the needle enters as a translator – not between therapist and client, but between mind and body.

The needle interrupts the loop.

It opens the gate between intellect and instinct.

And it reminds the body: You're allowed to let go now.

A Paradigm Shift

We're not here to throw away therapy. We're here to complete it.

To give it its missing limb: the body. The energy. The soul.

Psychology gave us language.

Acupuncture gives us release.

Together, they give us remembrance.

This is the beginning of the integration.

This is where healing becomes whole.

Chapter 2
The Body Remembers, But How?

"Your mind might forget. Your body never does."

Before a client says a single word, their body is already speaking.

Shoulders pulled up to the ears. Eyes darting. Legs that bounce restlessly. Or legs that freeze. Arms crossed protectively. A micro-holding in the breath. A slight tremor in the voice. A smile that doesn't quite meet the eyes.

These are not just nervous habits. They are soul signals.

As an acupuncturist, I learned to read these signs before I ever asked a question.

The body has its own language.

It doesn't speak in words.

It speaks in symptoms, sensations, and silence.

When a client says, "I don't remember what happened, but I feel it in my chest" – that is not a metaphor.

It is a literal expression of body-stored trauma – an intelligence that lives below cognition, beyond language, and within tissue.

To understand the missing link between psychology and acupuncture, we must first understand this:

The body does not forget what the mind can't hold.

And in many cases, the body is holding the entire story – waiting for someone to listen in its native tongue.

Psychology and the Somatic Blind Spot

Western psychology, for all its advances, often treats the body as a passive container for emotional experience – as if feelings happen in the mind, and the body just reacts.

But trauma researchers like Bessel van der Kolk, Stephen Porges, and Peter Levine have shown us the opposite:

The body is not the stage for trauma – it is the storyteller.

Through research into the nervous system, vagus nerve, fascia, and autonomic regulation, we now know:

- Emotional wounds manifest as muscular tension, gut disruption, chronic fatigue, and autoimmune dysregulation
- Traumatized bodies often stay locked in fight, flight, freeze, or fawn – even long after the threat is gone
- Talk therapy cannot reach these pre-verbal and sub-cortical patterns alone

This is where body-based modalities – especially acupuncture – become essential.

The Memory Systems of the Body

Let's explore three ways the body "remembers":

1. Neurological Memory - The Nervous System's Response Loop

Every trauma imprints a survival pattern.

Your nervous system learns what's "safe" or "dangerous" based on experience, not logic.

You might know someone loves you — but still flinch.

You might know you're not in danger — but still dissociate.

Acupuncture regulates the autonomic nervous system — especially via the vagus nerve and parasympathetic access points.

Calming the body's stress response allows it to repattern its reflexes.

2. Fascial & Muscular Memory – The Armored Body

The fascia is a web of connective tissue that wraps around every organ, muscle, and nerve.

When trauma occurs, the fascia contracts protectively — and often never fully relaxes.

Over time, this creates chronic holding patterns, emotional repression, and even energetic blockages along meridians.

Points like Gallbladder 21, Bladder 10, or Liver 14 are powerful portals into these patterns — not just physically, but emotionally.

3. Energetic Memory – The Meridian & Organ Intelligence

In Chinese medicine, every organ stores not just function, but emotion:

- Liver = anger, suppressed expression
- Lungs = grief, loss
- Kidneys = fear, ancestral memory
- Heart = betrayal, boundaries, heartbreak

Trauma doesn't just live in the brain.

It lives in the Liver Qi, the collapsed Lung meridian, the cold Kidneys of someone afraid to trust life again.

The needle is not just a tool – it's a translator.

It tells the body: I hear you now.

Polyvagal Theory Meets Meridian Theory

Let's bridge East and West for a moment.

Polyvagal theory gave us the language for what the ancients already knew: that the body stores memory, reacts faster than thought, and speaks in the dialect of survival. It teaches us that healing happens when the body enters the ventral vagal state – the zone of safety, connection, and regulation.

Fight. Flight. Freeze. Fawn. These are not just responses. They are relationships the body forms with life, based on past betrayal, neglect, or overwhelm.

Chinese medicine teaches us that healing occurs when Qi flows freely, unblocked by stagnation or excess.

What if these are saying the same thing… in different dialects?

Acupuncture stimulates vagal tone, releases emotional blockages, and restores Qi flow – which brings the body out of survival and into healing.

When you needle Stomach 36, you're not just boosting immunity – you're telling the body, "You're safe now. You can digest life again."

When you touch Kidney 6, you're not just aiding sleep – you're soothing generations of fear stored in the body's bones.

Western therapy may help someone understand why they're anxious. Acupuncture may help them feel less anxious. But what heals the part of them that is terrified to exist at all?

This is what the body remembers – and what the needle helps it finally release.

Needling the Nervous System

Acupuncture works beyond the verbal.

It reaches:

- The memories without words
- The sensations you couldn't explain
- The fears your mind forgot but your organs still carry

And most importantly, it reminds your body of something radical:

It doesn't have to be at war anymore.

When the Qi flows, the nervous system recalibrates.

When the meridians open, the story finds a way out.

When the body remembers safety – healing becomes inevitable.

When we work with the nervous system as oracle, every needle becomes a reverent question.

- Can you let go now?
- Can you feel safe here?
- Can you soften into presence?

Points along the Lung, Pericardium, Kidney, and Liver meridians are especially responsive to trauma work. But it is the intention behind the point that makes it medicine.

Paired with breath, voice, and guided invocation, needling becomes a ritual of rewiring.

I do not treat the nervous system. I honor it. I bow to its brilliance, its loyalty, its protection. Even its contractions are holy. They were built to keep the soul safe until it could return.

Now, it can.

The Nervous System Doesn't Need to Be Fixed. It Needs to Be Witnessed.

Let this chapter serve as a reframe:

You are not dysregulated. You are adaptive. You are not broken. You are brilliant. Your nervous system is not in the way of your healing. It is the way.

When we treat the body not as an obstacle but as an oracle, we begin to heal with reverence, not resistance.

We are entering a new era of healing — one that is multilingual.

Where therapists learn to feel.

Where acupuncturists learn to listen.

Where practitioners of all modalities learn to speak in the nervous system, meridian, and soul.

Psychology taught us to observe.

Acupuncture teaches us to embody.

Together, they bring us back to wholeness.

You are not broken.

You are not blocked.

You are holding something that your body never got to finish feeling.

And now, the body is ready.

And so are you.

And from here, all else becomes possible.

Case Example: The Man with the Silent Heart

Jason came to me for insomnia. He was a stoic high-performer. Never missed a day of work. "No trauma," he said.

But his pulse was wiry. His chest was tight. His eyes betrayed a grief his voice could not name.

I placed Heart 7 and Pericardium 6.

Within 15 minutes, tears streamed down his cheeks. He hadn't cried in over 20 years.

He said, "I don't know why I'm crying."

But his body knew.

The acupuncture point bypassed the mental gatekeeper.

The energy moved before the story surfaced.

Sometimes, the story is what follows the healing – not what precedes it.

Chapter 3
Energetics, Emotion, and the East

"Your emotions are not random. They are intelligent energy in motion – guided by ancient maps."

When people hear the word 'trauma,' they often think of events – war, abuse, accidents, heartbreak. But trauma is not the event itself. It is the imprint it leaves behind – a rupture in the body's sense of safety, wholeness, or belonging.

This imprint is not just psychological. It is energetic.

It moves like a current beneath the surface of the skin. It hides in the soft tissue. It loops in the meridians. It echoes in the breath, the womb, the spine. It leaves signatures not only on the brain, but on the soul's architecture.

In Psychology Acupuncture, we treat trauma not only as a memory but as a frequency. A vibration that can be listened to, honored, shifted – even alchemized.

In the West, we tend to see emotions as psychological phenomena.

In the East, emotions have always been understood as energetic movements – fluid forces that arise, circulate, and resolve through specific meridians and organ systems.

And in Chinese medicine, they are not just symbolic.

They are literal, diagnosable patterns affecting the body and soul.

What if your grief isn't just grief?

What if it's a signal from your Lung meridian – asking you to exhale what you were never taught to release?

Western medicine separates emotion from biology.

Eastern medicine never did.

Every tear, every panic attack, every tension in the neck is Qi in motion.

To heal, we must learn to speak the body's native language again.

And this is what the needle does:

- It doesn't just sedate or stimulate.
- It translates between feeling and form.
- It tells the organ: "You're not alone. You can exhale now."

This chapter explores how ancient Chinese medicine doesn't just describe emotion – it maps it.

Let's step into that map.

The Emotional Cartography of the Organs

Each organ system in Traditional Chinese Medicine (TCM) carries a physical function, an energetic role, and an emotional frequency. These are not poetic metaphors – they're diagnostic frameworks with thousands of years of case study.

Here are the five primary organ-emotion relationships:

LUNGS - Grief, Letting Go, Loss

- Element: Metal
- Season: Autumn

- Spirit: Po (corporeal soul)

The Lungs are the gatekeepers of inspiration and release.

When grief is unresolved, Lung Qi becomes stagnant or deficient.

Symptoms may include: shallow breathing, skin issues, melancholy, chronic colds, and fatigue.

Lung points help release held grief – especially LU 1, LU 7, and BL 13.

They also help with transitions – death, breakups, identity deaths – anything that asks us to let go.

Psychological Correlates: disenfranchised grief, hidden loss, unacknowledged endings

You don't "get over" grief. You exhale it. Again and again, through the Lungs.

HEART - Joy, Overwhelm, Heartbreak

- Element: Fire
- Season: Summer
- Spirit: Shen (consciousness/spirit)

The Heart governs consciousness, connection, and presence.

Emotional shock, betrayal, or heartbreak can disrupt the Shen, leading to anxiety, insomnia, or dissociation.

In Chinese medicine, the Heart "houses the spirit."

When the Heart is disturbed, we feel unanchored – even if life looks "fine" externally.

Key points: HT 7, PC 6, REN 14 – they soothe emotional chaos, reconnect you to your center.

Psychological Correlates: performative joy, fear of intimacy, emotional exhaustion

Your heartbreak isn't dysfunction – it's an invitation to reinhabit the Heart as sacred ground.

KIDNEYS - Fear, Ancestral Memory, Survival

- Element: Water
- Season: Winter
- Spirit: Zhi (willpower, destiny)

The Kidneys hold our Jing—the deepest well of life force. They store ancestral energy and primal fear.

When the Kidneys are weak or frozen in trauma:

- Fear becomes paralyzing
- Fatigue becomes existential
- The future feels unsafe

Kidney points, especially KI 3, KI 6, and BL 23, help recover lost willpower, access inner reserves, and heal inherited trauma.

Psychological Correlates: dissociation, existential fear, chronic overperformance

Not all your fear is yours. Some of it is passed down. The Kidney meridian knows the difference.

LIVER - Anger, Frustration, Suppressed Expression

- Element: Wood
- Season: Spring
- Spirit: Hun (ethereal soul, vision, dreams)

The Liver governs the free flow of Qi – physically, emotionally, and spiritually.

When emotions are repressed (especially anger), Liver Qi stagnates.

This leads to:

- PMS, migraines, digestive issues
- Irritability, resentment, depression
- Feeling "stuck" in life

Points like LIV 3, GB 34, and LIV 14 are used to release emotional congestion and restore momentum.

Psychological Correlates: suppressed rage, people-pleasing, learned helplessness

Anger is not bad. Suppressed anger is stagnation. The Liver helps you move it, not shame it.

SPLEEN – Worry, Overthinking, Self-Worth

- Element: Earth
- Season: Late Summer
- Spirit: Yi (intellect, thought)

The Spleen digests both food and thought.

It's where we process life – mentally, emotionally, and energetically.

Overthinking and worry weaken the Spleen, leading to:

- Fatigue, bloating, poor boundaries
- Anxious overcare, people-pleasing
- Lack of groundedness or self-trust

Key points: SP 6, ST 36, REN 12 – they help restore center and nourish self-worth.

Psychological Correlates: codependency, hyper-responsibility, self-neglect

When you feel scattered, don't just "calm down." Nourish your Earth. Come back to yourself.

Emotions Are Energetic Events

Here's the truth: Emotions are not pathology.

They are energetic weather patterns – meant to move through, not stay stuck in the body.

But when we suppress, bypass, or intellectualize them, they become:

- Illness
- Stagnation
- Misdiagnosed disorders

Chinese medicine treats emotions not as problems, but as patterns – each with a corresponding point, pulse quality, tongue pattern, and Qi expression.

You don't need to talk about the emotion to heal it.

You just need to release the energy beneath it.

This framework offers something most emotional models don't:

A physiological location for the emotional experience.

It helps clients:

- Feel their emotions in the body, not just describe them
- Move through stuck emotional patterns without needing a story
- Normalize emotional rhythms as natural, not pathological

It helps practitioners:

- Read symptoms as emotional signals
- Choose points based on emotional meridian blockages
- Hold emotional space with confidence and clarity

Bringing It All Together

You may not always know what a patient is feeling. But their body does.

The pulse will tell you. The channels will whisper. The organs will remember.

And when you listen—not just diagnostically, but emotionally—you become not just an acupuncturist. You become a translator of emotional truth.

This is the somatic language of the soul.

These aren't metaphors.

They're meridian realities.

- A woman suppressing her rage often presents with Liver stagnation, menstrual pain, jaw clenching, and rib-side distension.
- A man who won't allow himself to grieve holds a shallow Lung pulse, dry skin, and chronic upper back tension.
- A child overwhelmed with school pressure shows up with Spleen dampness, digestive upset, and mouth sores.

In Psychology Acupuncture, we use this ancient map to ask:

- What emotion has been repressed?
- What emotion has been unmetabolized?
- What organ has become the body's storage container for that weight?

And then, we use the needle to begin the transmutation.

This is the somatic language of truth. The organs don't lie.

Let us now enter the meridian of memory. And meet the parts of us that have been carrying the emotions we never let ourselves feel.

Where We Go From Here

You now understand the map.

You've seen how the body remembers, and how emotion travels through organs and meridians like ancient rivers.

But knowing the map is only the beginning.

In the next chapter, we'll explore how the needle becomes a compass – guiding us not just toward wellness, but toward wholeness.

Because healing isn't just about fixing what's broken.

It's about remembering what was always whole – and giving it a pathway home.

Part II

The Missing Link is You

Chapter 4
Holding Trauma in the Fascia

The first time I saw a patient begin to shake on the table, I thought it was a reaction to the needle. Then the tears came.

Then the memory.

And I realized I had touched more than a muscle or a meridian.

I had touched the **fascia**.

And the fascia had remembered.

In Chinese medicine, we are taught to think in meridians. In anatomy, we are taught to think in muscles.

But fascia? Fascia lives *between*.

It connects everything.

It is the body's interwoven matrix of memory, emotion, and protection.

Fascia doesn't just hold structure.

It holds a **story**.

And when it becomes rigid, it is often because the story was **never completed.**

If the organs are the keepers of emotion, the fascia is the **messenger**.

What Is Fascia?

Fascia is the connective tissue that wraps around every muscle, organ, nerve, and bone in your body. It is elastic, responsive, and highly innervated.

It communicates faster than the nervous system. It forms the structural integrity of our form. And it is deeply impacted by emotional trauma.

When we experience a threat, whether acute or prolonged, the fascia can freeze, harden, and adapt in protective patterns.

Over time, this creates:

- Chronic tightness or pain that doesn't resolve
- Emotional reactivity without cognitive cause
- Postural holding patterns rooted in experience

This is **not dysfunction**. It is an **intelligent adaptation**. But eventually, what once protected us begins to restrict us.

The Fascia as Emotional Memory

The body does not forget.

And fascia is one of its most loyal archivists.

We see this when:

- A woman begins to sob uncontrollably as Gallbladder 30 is needled, where she held the trauma of a sexual assault.
- A client begins to tremble at BL 52, where he carries the terror of childhood neglect.
- A young man starts to giggle, then cry at CV 6—the unwinding of years of holding his breath to avoid being noticed.

These aren't dramatic stories. They are **everyday miracles**.

The body is finally being given space to exhale what it has been holding.

How Needles Interact with Fascia

Acupuncture is not a superficial practice. Even at the thinnest layer, the needle touches fascia.

But certain techniques—and certain points—can access the deeper fascial matrix:

- **Threading techniques** along the myofascial planes create space.
- **Deeper insertions** in the hips, sacrum, or chest often access frozen emotions.
- **Shallow needling** can communicate with the Wei Qi and surface defenses, easing the fascia into release.

The key is not force.

It is an **invitation**.

The needle says: *It is safe to let go now.*

And if the fascia agrees, it will.

How to Recognize a Fascial Release

These are some signs I watch for:

- Sudden changes in temperature (sweating, chills)
- Twitching, trembling, or spontaneous movement
- Deep sighs, yawns, or softening of posture
- Emotional release without cognitive memory
- Vivid imagery or symbolic flashes

Sometimes, it happens fast.

Sometimes, it happens over time.

Sometimes, it doesn't happen until session seven.

But when it does?

You will feel it.

The pulse changes.

The energy shifts.

The entire room softens.

The Ethics of Unwinding

Just because the body can release doesn't mean it should release *right now*.

Trauma is sensitive, nonlinear, and layered. The fascia holds what it holds for a reason. And if we push too hard, too soon, we can **re-traumatize** rather than heal.

This is why pacing is sacred.

I often ask:

- "What are we making space for today?"
- "If your body could choose what to share, what would it want to show us?"
- "What feels tender right now?"

Let the *body* decide the sequence. You do not need to impress, diagnose, or deliver catharsis. You are there to **listen**.

Holding the Unwind

When the fascia releases, it can be disorienting. It can bring up imagery, sensations, or emotions that the patient does not have language for.

Here is how I hold that space:

- I don't ask for details.
- I guide them to stay present: "Can you breathe with that?"
- I validate the experience without interpretation.
- I track their breath and pulse to ensure grounding.

Often, I'll say:

"You don't need to make sense of it. Just stay with your body. It knows what it's doing."

And it always does.

Fascia as Spiritual Archive

I believe fascia doesn't just hold trauma.

It holds **lineage**.

I have had patients experience:

- Past-life recall during fascial release
- Ancestral grief emerging through somatic sensation
- Deep clarity around soul contracts, wounds, and timelines

You do not need to believe in mysticism to respect the mystery. The fascia holds more than the physical. It holds what the **spirit survived**.

And when we listen?

The body leads us back home.

Let your needles be gentle.

Let your questions be slow.

Let the fascia tell its story.

It has been waiting.

In Psychology Acupuncture, we treat fascia as **living tissue memory**. The needle doesn't just affect the muscle. It signals to the fascia: *you can let go now.*

We also explore the ethics of release. Because sometimes, what the fascia holds is **too big, too fast, too soon**. In Psychology Acupuncture, we learn to pace it. To listen. To create safety, not shock.

Your fascia is not just scar tissue. It's **a timeline**. A storage field. A spiritual boundary.

And when you learn to speak to it? You help the body *remember itself as a whole.*

The next time your patient cries 'for no reason' after a needle is placed—remember: That wasn't nothing. That was the **fascia finally telling the truth.**

Chapter 5
The Pulse That Speaks

In most traditional acupuncture programs, the pulse is taught as a diagnostic tool—a set of qualities and positions to memorize: slippery, wiry, thready, strong, deep, weak. One pulse for each organ. One finger for each position. We match the descriptions to conditions.

But the longer I listened, the more I realized:

The pulse doesn't just measure pathology. It is a **confession of truth.**

When read with presence and emotional attunement, the pulse becomes not just diagnostic—it becomes **dialogue**.

The Pulse as a Conversation

In Psychology Acupuncture, we don't just take the pulse. We **listen** to it. We attune to the frequency beneath the beat. We feel into what the patient isn't saying. Because sometimes, the pulse whispers what the voice cannot.

Each beat carries:

- Emotional residue
- Nervous system status
- Energetic reactivity
- Trauma imprints

I've held the wrist of someone who said they were fine, and felt an erratic, hidden panic. I've felt pulses drop out mid-beat when shame surfaced. I've tracked how the pulse in Heart position collapses when heartbreak is retold. The pulse reveals not just pathology, but *emotion in real time.*

Here's what I began to learn:

- A wiry Liver pulse can signal not just stress, but **repressed rage**
- A hollow Spleen pulse can mean more than deficiency—it often points to **chronic emotional self-neglect**
- A tight Kidney pulse may reflect **stored fear, especially around control, abandonment, or death**
- A full, bounding Heart pulse can reveal **anxiety masked as overperformance or people-pleasing**

I've felt pulses go into chaos after a needle touches truth.

I've felt them soften when the body finally says yes.

I've felt them vanish—momentarily—when trauma stirs.

This is not energetics.

This is **communication**.

The Three-Phase Pulse Read

In Psychology Acupuncture, I use a three-phase model:

1. Baseline Pulse

Before any conversation, I feel the pulse in silence. This tells me the *starting point*.

- Are they grounded?
- Are they fragmented?
- Is their Shen (spirit) present?

I note speed, strength, shape, and spirit.

2. Relational Pulse

As we begin the inquiry, I place my fingers on the pulse again. I watch what changes *in real time* as they speak.

- Does the Liver pulse rise when they talk about their job?
- Does the Heart pulse flutter when their ex is mentioned?
- Does the Kidney pulse tighten when we ask about rest or control?

This helps me identify what topics **dysregulate** them—even if they seem composed on the outside.

3. Post-Needle Pulse

After point insertion, I revisit the pulse. This is where the story shifts.

- Does the pulse slow down?
- Does the Spleen position open?
- Does the tension dissipate?

Sometimes, a single point will restore coherence across the entire system. Other times, the pulse tells me: not today. The body isn't ready.

Reading for Emotion, Not Just Syndrome

The pulse doesn't only tell me if the Liver is excessive or the Spleen is deficient. It tells me:

- Where they're holding grief
- Whether their anger is outward or internalized
- If their Shen is fractured or full
- Whether their willpower is online

When you read the pulse through this lens, it becomes a **living, feeling document**. You begin to sense:

- The collapse in the Lung pulse of a client who hasn't cried in years
- The manic flutter in the Heart pulse of someone masking anxiety with productivity
- The slow, thready Kidney pulse of someone whose trauma has drained their reserves

This is where the pulse stops being diagnostic. And becomes **intimate**.

How the Pulse Guides Treatment

I don't always start with symptoms. I start with the **pulse**.

Because if the pulse is wiry but the words are calm, I know we're not treating what they think we are.

If the pulse is erratic when they talk about their mother, I know that's the portal.

If the pulse disappears when grief is mentioned, I know to tread slowly, gently.

The pulse isn't a static measurement. It's a **living mirror**.

And when I let it guide me, the treatment becomes more precise, more honest, more effective.

Building the Skill of Pulse Listening

Reading the pulse this way requires:

- Stillness
- Practice
- Presence

- Emotional neutrality

You must be:

- Grounded in your own nervous system
- Willing to feel what your patient cannot say
- Clear enough to separate your intuition from projection
- This is not "intuitive" work. It is **trained sensitivity**.
- And the more you practice, the more the pulse speaks.

When the Pulse Shifts, the Field Shifts

The moment I know something has landed is when the pulse changes.

- The quality softens.
- The Shen becomes visible.
- The body says: *yes*.

It's a quiet miracle. But it changes everything.

You don't need your client to tell you they've shifted.

You'll feel it in your fingers.

Some of the most powerful validations I've received in session haven't been from a patient's words—they've been from their pulse returning to harmony.

The body always tells you when it's ready. The pulse tells you when it's safe.

And when can you feel that? You're not just treating a condition. You're walking beside someone as they come back to life.

Chapter 6
The Needles As Oracle

"It was never just a needle. It was always a message."

The Needle Doesn't Just Treat – It Translates

For centuries, acupuncture has been used to:

- Stimulate healing
- Move Qi
- Relieve symptoms

But in the hands of an attuned practitioner, the needle becomes something more:

- A **mirror**
- A **messenger**
- A **medium** between the seen and unseen

There is a moment in the session that I have come to revere. It doesn't happen every time, and it can never be forced.

It is the moment when the needle, placed with precision and presence, unlocks the story the body has been waiting to tell.

Sometimes it arrives as a sudden memory.

Sometimes, as a flood of emotion, tears, or a visceral sigh.

Sometimes, as silence—the kind so full it hums.

This is not a coincidence. It is resonance.

It is the sacred language of the subconscious answering back.

A needle is more than a tool for physical healing. In the right hands, it becomes a compass. A key. A spell. When placed with intention, ritual, and soul awareness, a needle does more than shift qi — it opens memory.

This is not esoteric fantasy. It is a clinical mystery.

I have watched as a client, when needled at a soul acupoint, suddenly recalled the exact moment they chose to abandon their voice at five years old. I have seen ancestral sorrow release from the womb, tremble through the legs, and finally leave with an exhale.

In ancient Taoist practice, acupuncture wasn't just about health. It was **divinatory**. **Spiritual**. Even **oracular**.

The body was seen as a cosmic map, and the meridians were channels not just of Qi, but of **memory, emotion, and soul wisdom**.

And the practitioner? Not just a technician.

But an **interpreter of energy**. A **listener** of what the body was too wise to verbalize.

The body does not lie. The body does not forget. And when we listen with sacred attention, the body becomes the bridge between the mind and the soul.

I still remember the moment I stopped treating points as protocols.

I was sitting with a client, chart in hand, ready to follow the classic pattern: Liver Qi stagnation, hormonal imbalance, emotional stress. The prescription was obvious.

But something in my gut whispered: *Not yet.* My hand hovered, intuitively drawn to a point I rarely used in this context —

Pericardium 8. It wasn't in the books for hormone regulation, but my body knew.

Within seconds of needling, the client burst into tears. "I don't know what's happening," she said. "I just remembered something I haven't thought about in 20 years."

That moment changed everything.

The needle wasn't just healing her hormones. It was unlocking a memory, a message, a moment in time her body was finally ready to reclaim.

A New Framework Begins

This chapter is not about dismissing psychology or abandoning acupuncture. It is about reclaiming what both have forgotten: that true healing requires the sacred.

In the chapters ahead, you will meet the Soul Acupoints. You will learn the AcuRitual. You will witness stories of healing that defy diagnosis. But first, you must understand: The mind cannot be healed without the body. The body cannot be healed without the soul. And the soul cannot be healed without being remembered.

This is the medicine that has been missing. Until now.

Case Example: The Girl with the Disconnected Voice

Sarah was 19 and had lost her voice — literally. Doctors said it was anxiety. Her vocal cords were healthy. Her tests were normal.

But she hadn't spoken in weeks.

She sat silently across from me. Her eyes were hollow, and her energy had collapsed.

I felt drawn to **Kidney 6**, **Lung 7**, and **Ren 22**. But more than that, I felt drawn to her *Po* – the **corporeal soul** that resides in the Lungs.

After placing the needles, she trembled. Her throat flushed pink. Tears rolled down her cheeks. And then, for the first time in over a month, she whispered:

"I didn't want to lie anymore."

She hadn't lost her voice. She had silenced it – to survive a betrayal she couldn't yet speak of.

The needle didn't "fix" her. It opened the door to the **truth** her body had been guarding.

Case Example: The Woman with "No Anger"

Angela had no anger. She said it with a smile: "I just don't get mad. "Her pulse was wiry. Her Liver was screaming.

She suffered from migraines, IBS, and a stuck career.

I placed **Liver 3**, **Gallbladder 34**, and **Pericardium 8**. After a few minutes, her body started trembling. She whispered, "I think I've been swallowing my truth for years."

She didn't need a rage ritual. She needed a **release valve**.

Within a few sessions, her headaches disappeared. Her digestion improved. And – for the first time in 12 years – she asked for a raise.

Acupuncture didn't teach her to be angry. It gave her permission to feel again.

Protocol vs. Presence

There is nothing wrong with protocols. They are scaffolding. Foundation. Structure.

But something happens when a practitioner shifts from:

- "What points match the pattern?" to
- "What is the body saying — and what point wants to speak next?"

You move from **thinking** to **listening**. From **treating** to **translating**. From **practicing medicine** to **channeling medicine**.

This shift is subtle — but sacred. And it changes everything.

The Body as Oracle, the Practitioner as Channel

The meridians are not mechanical. They are **living rivers** of information — emotional, ancestral, spiritual.

Each needle placed is a **conversation**:

- You ask a question
- The body responds
- The energy shifts
- A story emerges

This is why two clients with the "same pattern" will respond completely differently to the same points.

Because their bodies carry **different messages**, **different timelines, different soul contracts**.

You are not treating a diagnosis. You are entering a dialogue.

And the needle? It is the **ink** in which that dialogue is written.

Chapter 7
Psychology Acupuncture – A New Modality

"Where the mind meets the meridian, healing remembers how to move."

There comes a point in every healing path where the modalities begin to blur.

Is it trauma or Qi stagnation? Is it a cognitive distortion or a Kidney deficiency? Is it emotional suppression or liver heat rising?

The answer is: *yes*.

Because the separation between **psychology** and **acupuncture** was never natural. It was imposed. It was the result of a medical model that divided mind from body, science from spirit, healer from patient.

But deep healing requires **integration**. **Psychology Acupuncture** is that integration.

It's not just combining two fields. It's **reweaving the wholeness** they both came from.

What Is Psychology Acupuncture?

Psychology Acupuncture is the intentional blending of:

- **Clinical psychological insight**
- **Traditional Chinese medicine & acupuncture**
- **Energetic and somatic intelligence**

- **Soul-level, multidimensional awareness**

It's a **multilingual healing method** that allows emotional, mental, energetic, and ancestral trauma to be addressed – not separately, but **simultaneously**.

In a Psychology Acupuncture session, you are not only:

- Treating the nervous system
- Moving stagnant Qi
- Supporting the organs
- Validating the emotional body

You are **allowing all parts of the self** – psyche, soma, spirit – to come into coherence.

The Four Pillars of Psychology Acupuncture

1. Emotional Diagnosis

Rather than simply diagnosing by symptoms, we ask:

- *What unprocessed emotion is stored here?*
- *What organ system or meridian is trying to speak?*
- *What inner child, archetype, or wound is activated?*

This is not emotional speculation – it is a **clinical attunement to the body's emotional language**, based in both TCM and trauma psychology.

2. Meridian-Based Emotional Mapping

Each acupuncture point is understood not just physiologically, but **psychoenergetically**.

Examples:

- **SP 6** to anchor excessive worry and support self-worth
- **LIV 14** to release suppressed grief masked as rage
- **PC 7** to resolve betrayal trauma and restore trust

Points are chosen not to "fix" a symptom, but to **facilitate emotional and energetic resolution**.

3. Somatic and Nervous System Integration

Trauma is processed **bottom-up**: through the body first, not the mind.

We use acupuncture to:

- Exit chronic sympathetic survival states
- Activate the vagus nerve
- Restore safe embodiment
- Integrate trauma *without re-traumatizing*

The goal is not emotional catharsis – it is **nervous system safety** and **energetic recalibration**.

4. Soul-Centered Listening

Every session includes space for the client's:

- Inner knowing
- Dreams, visions, and ancestral memories
- Archetypes, soul contracts, karmic patterns

The practitioner becomes a **channel**, not just a clinician – allowing the body's wisdom to guide the session in co-creation.

Why This Modality Matters Now

The collective is experiencing:

- Widespread trauma
- Fragmented identity
- Burnout from cognitive overload
- Skepticism toward spiritual bypass

Clients are not just looking for healing – they're looking for **truth**. And truth lives **in the body**.

Psychology Acupuncture offers:

- A grounded alternative to spiritual "fluff"
- A heart-centered complement to clinical therapy
- A bridge for those who feel broken by systems and unseen by science

This is medicine for the **modern mystic**. This is healing for the **whole human**.

Oracular Acupuncture Is Not Woo – It's Ancient

In the earliest lineages of Chinese medicine:

- Practitioners meditated for hours before sessions
- Needles were used during **astrological alignments**
- The **spirit of each point** was invoked before needling

This wasn't superstition. It was **reverence**.

They knew what modern science is just beginning to rediscover:

- That every cell holds memory
- That the body's energy field carries past and future timelines
- That healing isn't linear – it's **layered, multidimensional, and often miraculous**

You don't need to choose between **evidence-based practice** and **intuitive medicine**.The future of healing is **hybrid**.

Healing at the Frequency Level

To release trauma from the energy field, the practitioner must:

1. Recognize the imprint (diagnose beyond symptoms)
2. Honor the protective role it played (witness without force)
3. Introduce a new frequency (through ritual, needle, breath, presence)

Points like Pericardium 6, Kidney 3, Liver 14, and REN 17 become oracular when approached this way.

But even more important than the points are the practitioner's presence, permission, and prayer.

This is not about "fixing" the trauma. This is about transforming it into wisdom.

So how does this all work?

How do you bring soul acupoints, energetic imprints, nervous system tracking, and ceremony together in a session, and still hold the clinical clarity that makes a client feel safe?

This chapter is where theory becomes practice. Where the mystical meets the method. Psychology Acupuncture is not a rigid protocol — it is a flexible ritual technology. But it has rhythm, structure, and deep internal logic.

Intuitive Point Selection: A Sacred Skill

You might be wondering:

- *How do I trust that intuitive nudge?*

- *What if I get it wrong?*
- *What if it's just my imagination?*

Here's the truth: **intuition is a muscle**. It sharpens with practice, presence, and humility.

Here are a few ways it speaks:

- A **heat** in your hand when you hover over a point
- A **vision** or word that arises uninvited
- A **tingle, tightness**, or **resonance** in your own body
- A **memory** that doesn't feel like yours, but belongs to the client

These are not random. They are **energetic invitations**. You don't need to explain them to anyone else – only honor them.

Over time, you begin to learn that **the point chooses you as much as you choose it**.

Integration Practice: Listening Before You Needle

Before your next session, try this:

1. Sit quietly with the client's energy
2. Forget the diagnosis
3. Place one hand over your own heart
4. Ask silently:

What does this body want to say? What point wants to speak today?

4. Breathe. Listen. Feel.
5. Choose the point that **responds** – not just the one that makes "sense"

You are not guessing. You are remembering.

You Are the Missing Link

This chapter is not about giving up your knowledge. It's about **reclaiming your knowing**.

You were not trained to be a robot. You were born to be a **bridge** – between science and spirit, body and soul, symptom and story.

The needle is your pen. The meridian is the sentence. The body is the poem.

And you? You are the oracle.

The 7 Soul Acupoints and the Map to Inner Remembrance

After the collapse, something new emerged. Not just a theory. Not just a method. But a map.

It came in dreams, in ceremony, in the silent language of the body. Seven gates – not strictly anatomical, but archetypal. Energetic. Mythic.

Each of these points carried a story. A wound. A medicine.

This chapter offers you the **Soul Acupoints**: the energetic coordinates of the human experience, seen through the eyes of Psychology Acupuncture.

The Soul Speaks in Symbols

When I work with clients, I don't only listen to what they say. I listen to where their grief lives. I watch where the breath gets caught. I feel the contraction behind their diagnosis.

These seven Soul Acupoints emerged from thousands of sacred sessions. They are a living map — meant to guide you inward, not to bind you outward.

They invite you to ask not just "What's wrong with me?" but "What part of me is ready to be reclaimed?"

1. The Point of Exile

Location: Below the collarbone (LU 1 region)

Wound: "I don't belong."

Medicine: Grounding, breath, ancestral reconnection

Use for: Disconnection, identity loss, grief, spiritual isolation

Ritual Phrase: *"With this breath, I return to the Earth of my body. I belong."*

2. The Point of Betrayal

Location: Center of sternum (REN 17 / Pericardium Gate)

Wound: "I can't trust."

Medicine: Softening the heart wall, receiving love

Use for: Heartbreak, abandonment, spiritual betrayal

Ritual Phrase: *"Even in betrayal, my heart remains sacred."*

3. The Point of Suppression

Location: Throat center (Ren 22 / Window of the Sky)

Wound: "My truth is dangerous."

Medicine: Reclaiming voice and visibility

Use for: Witch wounds, performance fear, expression block

Ritual Phrase: *"My voice is a sacred instrument of remembrance."*

4. The Point of Guilt

Location: Solar plexus (REN 12)

Wound: "I am responsible for their pain."

Medicine: Boundary restoration, personal sovereignty

Use for: Codependency, people-pleasing, ancestral guilt

Ritual Phrase: *"I release what was never mine to carry."*

5. The Point of Self-Rejection

Location: Lower abdomen/womb space (REN 4)

Wound: "Something in me is wrong."

Medicine: Creative innocence, inner child healing

Use for: Shame, fertility trauma, sexual repression, creative blocks

Ritual Phrase: *"I come home to the parts I once abandoned."*

6. The Point of Collapse

Location: Kidney area (KID 3 or BL 23)

Wound: "I'm not safe in my body."

Medicine: Safety, grounding, trauma regulation

Use for: Freeze response, chronic fear, adrenal fatigue

Ritual Phrase: *"It is now safe to be here. My body is my anchor."*

7. The Point of Destiny

Location: Third eye / Yintang

Wound: "I don't know who I am."

Medicine: Soul vision, mission clarity, intuitive awakening

Use for: Identity crisis, spiritual stagnation, disconnection from purpose

Ritual Phrase: *"I remember who I am across lifetimes."*

The Psychology Acupuncture AcuRitual

While these points can be used in traditional sessions, their true power awakens when paired with sacred presence.

The **AcuRitual** is a ceremonial approach that blends:

- Intuitive diagnosis
- Needle as invocation
- Visualization and guided breath
- Aromatic or vibrational medicine
- Dialogue with the wounded archetype

Here, the practitioner becomes a priestess. The needle becomes a wand. The session becomes a rite of passage.

These points are not mine to own. They are ours to remember.

As you explore them – in clients, in yourself – allow your body to speak. You may discover new variations. You may hear whispers from your lineage. You may meet archetypes not yet written.

Good. This framework is living. You are not here to memorize it. You are here to animate it.

Now that you've received the map, the journey begins.

Where We Go From Here

Now that the foundation is laid, the question becomes:

How does this look in practice?

How do we invite the soul into the session?

How do we work with timelines, karma, betrayal, embodiment, and dreamwork?

In the next chapter, we step beyond modality and into **mystery** – where healing becomes a **soul ceremony**.

Because now that you've remembered the method, you're ready to remember **who you are when you use it**.

Step 1: The Listening Field

Before any questions are asked, before pulse or tongue is observed, I enter the field of **energetic listening**.

This means dropping in. Grounding. Opening my own body as a tuning fork for truth.

Clients often begin with a story. But I'm listening beneath the story.

- **What does their posture say before they speak?**
- **What is happening in the pulse before they describe a symptom?**
- **What does their breath do when I ask them to close their eyes?**

This is a soul diagnosis. Not to fix, but to *feel for the invitation.*

This includes:

- Pulse dynamics (speed, quality, responsiveness)
- Shen observation (eye clarity, voice tone, spirit presence)
- Body language (fidgeting, stillness, freeze response)
- Somatic intuition (what I feel in *my* body in their presence)
- Protective patterning (distraction, deflection, smile masking)

Energetic reading is **not analysis**. It is a deep, neutral observation.

Before they speak, I've already adjusted my tone, my breathing, and my nervous system to meet them where they are.

The container begins *before* the session.

It is made of nervous system coherence, not words.

From here, I begin to sense which **Soul Acupoints** may be calling for activation.

Step 2: Somatic Inquiry (Relational Dialogue)

Once the field is attuned and the pulse is taken, I move into gentle dialogue.But unlike traditional talk therapy, these questions are **rooted in the body**, not the narrative.

Instead of:

- "Why do you think that happened?"
- I ask:
- "Where do you feel that in your body right now?"
- Instead of:
- "What do you want to change?"
- I ask:

- "If your body could speak, what would it say about this?"
- This phase prioritizes:
- **Localization:** Mapping sensation to emotion to point selection.
- **Permission:** Letting the client guide the depth. Never forcing.
- **Containment:** Watching for overwhelm or dissociation and slowing the pace accordingly.

This is *not* about intellectual insight. It is about allowing the body to speak in sensation, image, and intuition.

Sometimes, we never get to needles. Because what needed to shift, already did.

But most often, this inquiry reveals the exact pathway the needle is meant to follow.

Step 3: The Soul Mapping

Together, we track the issue across three layers:

1. Psychological – thoughts, emotions, identity
2. Somatic – where it lives in the body
3. Energetic – frequency, archetype, memory

Using these three lenses, I determine which Soul Acupoints and classical points to activate.

I also choose which tools will be used:

- Needling
- Moxa
- Breath and visualization

Each session becomes a **ceremony of recalibration**.

Step 4: The AcuRitual Begins

The AcuRitual is what makes this work different.

We begin with breath. Then the intention. Then the needle – placed not just with skill, but with presence.

At each Soul Acupoint, I whisper the client's chosen phrase. Or I ask them to repeat it as I place the needle:

"It is now safe to be here."

"I release what was never mine."

"I remember who I am."

Then we rest. Sometimes with sound. Sometimes in silence. Always in the field of remembrance.

Step 5: Integration and Revelation

After needles are removed, we do not rush. This is where **gold returns to the surface.**

- What did you feel?
- What memory or image arose?
- What part of you returned?

Often, this is when the client receives a breakthrough. A vision. A message. A release.

I record these. I name them. I anchor them. Because this is not just symptom relief – this is **soul retrieval**.

What a Client Might Say:

- "I didn't know how much I was holding."
- "I felt my grandmother with me."
- "It's like something left me — in a good way."
- "That was a ceremony. Not a session."

This is what happens when you treat the body as a temple. When you see the soul, not just the symptoms.

What Happens After the Soul Returns?

Clients often report:

- Renewed clarity or purpose
- Spontaneous lifestyle changes
- Shedding of old identities
- Unexplainable sense of "coming home"
- Emotional detox or subtle grief as they re-inhabit the body

This is not a coincidence.

It's the **return of their original blueprint**.

And it often begins not with a breakthrough, but with a **needle, placed with love**, at the right moment, in the right portal.

The Witch Doctor Way

You do not need to be a shaman or mystic to practice this. You need only remember:

- The body already knows.
- The soul already remembers.
- The needle, with reverence, reveals the way.

This method cannot be performed. It must be **embodied**.

It requires:

- Nervous system regulation
- Stillness without withdrawal
- Presence without performance
- Boundaries without rigidity

You are not healing them. You are creating the space where their body can remember *how* to heal.

What makes this method work is not the point prescription.

It is your ability to hold **attuned neutrality** while the story unfolds.

You must become the medicine your client's body has never experienced before

In the next chapter, we will move deeper into collective and ancestral trauma — and how Psychology Acupuncture allows us to work with the invisible weight we carry.

But for now, take a breath. Feel your own body.

That is the field we work in. That is the field that remembers you.

You are not just treating symptoms.

You are witnessing **soul reassembly**.

You are midwifing **remembrance**.

Your clients may not have the words.

But their bodies will say:

Thank you. I feel more like myself than I have in years.

And you'll know: That part of them, the one they thought they lost, has come home.

Chapter 8
The Soul in the Session

"The body holds the map. The needle opens the portal. The soul remembers the way home."

There comes a moment in the healing journey – often quiet, unplanned – when you realize:

This isn't just about symptoms anymore.

This is about the soul.

What we thought was anxiety… was a karmic loop.

What we thought was chronic pain… was ungrieved ancestral grief.

What we thought was resistance… was a soul fragment that hadn't returned yet.

Not all trauma is personal. Some of it is collective. Some of it is inherited. Some of it is karmic.

- The woman who fears being seen but has no memory of harm – until she sees a vision of herself burned at the stake.
- The man who cannot rest unless he is overworking, until he feels the energy of generations who survived by labor.
- The child born to a mother who was grieving – and now lives with a grief that was never theirs to begin with.
- Trauma can enter the system through:
- Personal experiences
- Intergenerational memory
- Ancestral DNA and epigenetics

- Past life recall or karmic residue
- Collective field resonance (e.g., cultural trauma, war, diaspora)

This is why trauma work must evolve. It is not just about what happened *to* us. It is about what lives *in* us – even if we didn't choose it.

In this chapter, we go deeper.

Into the soul field.

Into the unseen dimensions where real healing begins.

Because a true healing session doesn't just balance energy.

It retrieves what was lost.

It completes what was unfinished.

It remembers what was once forgotten.

The Body is the Bridge

The mind may forget. The body does not.

That is why trauma often bypasses logic. You can understand why something happened and still feel panic in your chest, numbness in your belly, or grief in your bones. Because the body holds what the mind cannot.

This is where energetic healing becomes vital. Talk therapy may bring insight. But acupuncture brings release. It gives the body a new story. A new frequency to hold.

In Psychology Acupuncture, we use the body as a bridge between the conscious self and the soul imprint. The needle, placed with intention and reverence, becomes a tuning fork – shifting the frequency of the imprint from survival to sovereignty.

The Invisible Signature of Trauma

I've seen trauma show up in:

- A voice that won't speak
- A womb that won't conceive
- A jaw that can't unclench
- A dream that repeats like a ritual

These are not random symptoms. They are soul signals.

One client came in with recurring neck tension. No physical injury. No emotional insight. But every time I palpated the area, she would freeze. Her breath would stop. Her pupils would dilate.

Eventually, during a treatment, she wept and said, "I don't think I was allowed to say no."

No memory. Just a knowing.

This is how energetic trauma reveals itself – not always as memory, but as *resonance.*

Collective Trauma Lives in the Field

Some of the heaviest burdens we carry are not ours. And yet, they live in our blood, our bones, our dreams.

A woman who fears her own power but cannot trace the source. A man who grieves a loss that never happened in his lifetime. A child born into silence, already carrying shame that was never theirs.

This is the domain of **collective, ancestral, and karmic trauma** – energetic imprints that predate our individual story but continue to shape our nervous system, identity, and expression.

Psychology Acupuncture gives us tools to work in this space with precision, reverence, and soul remembrance.

We are not separate from the collective. We breathe in its memory. We inherit its fear. We move through its unresolved grief.

Wars. Colonization. Genocide. Religious persecution. Diaspora. Suppression of the feminine. Erasure of indigenous knowledge. These are not just historical facts. They are living frequencies – stored in the collective body and echoed in our personal symptoms.

When a client presents with emotional patterns that defy individual experience – such as unexplained terror, shame without origin, or chronic existential dread – we listen for the collective imprint.

Needles placed at Soul Acupoints (especially the Point of Collapse and Point of Exile) can unlock memories not of this life, but of a collective wound.

Ancestral Memory in the Body

Our ancestors passed down more than DNA. They passed down unresolved stories, suppressed truths, and unfinished grief.

Science calls this **epigenetics**. Spirit calls it **ancestral inheritance**.

Psychology Acupuncture meets both.

In session, a client may begin to cry for a grandmother they never met. They may feel the weight of generations of women silenced. They may suddenly speak words in a language they've never studied.

This is the body remembering.

Points along the Kidney, Liver, and Pericardium meridians – when approached ceremonially – become channels for ancestral healing.

Ritual phrases like:

- "I witness you now."
- "What was buried will now be honored."
- "Your healing is my liberation."

...can activate deep releases that ripple through timelines.

Karmic Threads and Soul Contracts

Sometimes, what we carry is older than ancestry. It is **karmic** – chosen by the soul for healing, evolution, or resolution.

This includes:

- Repeating relationship patterns
- Chronic blocks that persist despite deep work
- Fears or skills that appear with no logical source

Through intuitive listening and needle invocation, we can open the Akashic body – the energetic layer where soul contracts live.

The Point of Destiny and Point of Betrayal are especially potent in karmic work.

Clients often receive visions, past life downloads, or sudden clarity about current entanglements.

We do not force these experiences. We create the **conditions of sacred safety** for them to emerge.

The Soul Is Not a Metaphor

In Psychology Acupuncture, the soul is not a poetic idea. It is a *living intelligence* – multidimensional, cyclical, encoded in the meridians and spirit systems of Chinese medicine.

In Taoist Five-Spirit theory, every organ houses a spiritual aspect:

Organ	**Spirit**	**Function**
Heart	Shen	Consciousness, Presence
Liver	Hun	Vision, Imagination, Destiny
Lung	Po	Instinct, Grief, Corporeal Memory
Spleen	Yi	Intellect, Integration
Kidney	Zhi	Willpower, Soul Memory, Survival Blueprint

Together, they form a **spirit constellation**. When one or more are fragmented, we see it not only in the pulse, but in the soul's ability to feel *here, safe, clear, connected.*

Trauma isn't just what happened. Trauma is the moment the **Shen left the body** to survive.

Soul Fragmentation & Retrieval

Soul fragmentation happens in moments of overwhelm, betrayal, violence, or grief – when staying fully embodied would have been too dangerous.

It shows up in:

- Emotional numbness
- Memory blanks
- Dissociation
- Feeling "off" or "not all here"
- Chronic disempowerment or confusion
- Therapy breakthroughs that don't "stick"

These aren't mental health issues alone. They are **soul health** issues. And the body often knows it before the mind does.

When the Hun cannot envision, depression settles. When the Po is suppressed, grief calcifies. When the Zhi is weakened, fear becomes fate.

How the Needle Facilitates Soul Return

Needles placed with soul-level intention can:

- Call back fragments of self that dissociated
- Stabilize the field after emotional or psychic rupture
- Help complete a karmic memory held in the tissues
- Invite ancestral integration through the Po or Zhi
- Open access to inner guidance via the Hun or Shen

Examples:

- **BL 42 (Po Hu - Door of the Corporeal Soul)** — for releasing unprocessed grief and calling back body wisdom
- **LIV 8 (Qu Quan - Spring at the Crook)** — for reintegrating vision, forgotten desires, inner child dreams
- **KD 6 (Zhao Hai - Shining Sea)** — to open soul memory through the Zhi and dream pathways
- **HT 7 (Shen Men - Spirit Gate)** — to re-anchor presence after trauma or heartbreak

You're not just needling a point. You're opening a door. And the soul — when invited gently — walks through.

Working with Dreams, Visions & Nonlinear Guidance

In Psychology Acupuncture, sessions may include:

- Client's recurring dreams
- Sudden memories or visions during the session
- Ancestral presences or energetic messages
- Intuitive images that arise in you, the practitioner

These are not distractions. They are **data** — soul data. They tell us what's being metabolized beneath cognition.

You don't need to interpret everything. You just need to hold space.

Ask:

- *"What does this image want you to remember?"*
- *"If your body were telling a story, what chapter is this?"*
- *"What wants to come home today?"*

The Alchemy of Witnessing

In the old traditions, the wound was not shameful. It was sacred. It marked the place where the initiate had met the edge of life and returned with vision.

Your trauma is not your identity. But it *is* your portal.

In the temple of the body, we do not extract pain. We listen to it. We translate it. We offer it new form.

Through Psychology Acupuncture, trauma becomes less of a scar and more of a song.

You are not broken. You are encoded.

And healing is not erasure. It is **remembrance**.

Chapter 9
Trauma Is Not A Trend – It's A Somatic War

We are living in a time when trauma is trending.

It has become a buzzword in marketing, a hook in influencer content, a brand identity in spiritual circles.

#trauma

#nervoussystemhealing

#innerchildwork

And while it is a miracle that we are finally naming our pain, we must remember:

Trauma is not an aesthetic.

Trauma is not content.

Trauma is a somatic war.

It is not just what happened to you.

It is what didn't finish happening.

The scream that got swallowed.

The shaking that never discharged.

The grief that calcified behind the eyes.

Trauma is not only in the memory.

It's in the fascia.

The pulse.

The pericardium.

The field.

When we treat trauma as a trend, we cheapen the sacred process of integration.

We pathologize normal responses to abnormal circumstances.

We confuse emotional literacy with emotional performance. And when it becomes performance, we risk mistaking awareness for integration.

The Danger of Trauma Performance

In Psychology Acupuncture, trauma is not something to be flaunted. It is something to be felt, honored, and slowly alchemized.

This is not about gatekeeping.

It's about guardianship.

There is a difference between being trauma-informed and being trauma-performative.

The performative path looks like:

- Speaking the language but bypassing the body
- Using trauma as identity rather than inquiry
- Making healing about aesthetics, not attunement
- Becoming addicted to diagnosis instead of curiosity
- This kind of performance keeps the story alive without resolution.

It floods the nervous system with activation but offers no repair.

Because when trauma becomes branding, the body becomes performance. But when trauma is honored as sacred wound-work, the body becomes altar.

Awareness without containment is just reactivation.

What the Body Needs Instead

The body doesn't want your insight.

It doesn't need poetic captions.

It doesn't care how many workshops you've attended.

It wants:

- Rhythm
- Safety
- Co-regulation
- Space to discharge

The body wants to finish the thing it never got to finish.

That means shaking, crying, melting, sighing.

That means needing someone to say:

"You're safe. I'm here. Let it move."

That is what we do with Psychology Acupuncture.

We don't just talk about trauma.

We touch it.

We listen to it.

We mirror it back in silence.

The Practitioner's Responsibility

In this work, we must be trauma-literate and trauma-humble.

We must:

- Know our own trauma so we don't project it
- Regulate ourselves before co-regulating a client
- Stop chasing catharsis
- Learn when to slow down
- Recognize the difference between release and re-traumatization

We do not poke at wounds.

We wait until the body shows us it is ready.

Just because a client can talk about something doesn't mean they are ready to move it.

We must stop conflating language with readiness.

Healing is Slow. Sacred. Somatic.

True healing is not glamorous.

It's not viral.

It's often quiet.

It happens in sessions no one sees.

It happens in the silence between the needle and the tears.

Healing looks like:

- Breathing for the first time in years
- Realizing your anger is sacred
- Grieving the mother you never had
- Saying no without guilt
- Choosing rest without collapse

These are not moments for the camera.

They are moments for the altar.

You Are the Field, Not the Fix

When we work with trauma, we do not fix.

We do not heal.

We hold.

We become the regulated field that the nervous system never had.

We say, through tone and pulse and presence:

"You are safe to remember now."

That is the real work.

That is what trauma requires.

Not performance.

But presence.

Not branding.

But boundaries.

Not aesthetics.

But attunement.

Let the Somatic War End

Your client's body is not broken.

It is brilliant.

It adapted.

It protected.

It survived.

But it does not want to keep surviving.

It wants to rest.

It wants to be completed.

It wants to return.

Our job is to stop making trauma the center of attention.

And start making the body the center of trust.

Let the war end.

Let the nervous system lead.

Let the needle speak.

Because trauma is not a trend.

It is a sacred wound that deserves reverence, not reposts.

And healing is not a brand.

It is a reclamation.

Let's stop selling trauma.

Let's start witnessing it.

Let's offer the body a safe place to remember who it was before the war—and who it still has the power to become.

Let us treat it that way.

Part III

Reclaiming the Sacred Healer Within

Chapter 10
From Practitioner to Priestess

"You didn't come here to hide behind credentials. You came here to carry medicine only your soul remembers."

Let's speak a sacred truth:

You didn't come here to repeat what's been taught. You came here to **remember what was forgotten.**

You came to collapse false authority. You came to reclaim the healer who doesn't just treat —**she initiates, she channels, she changes the room when she walks in.**

There comes a turning point in every medicine carrier's life — when the method alone is no longer enough. When the work begins to ask more of you—not more knowledge, not more tools.

But more **truth**.

That moment isn't burnout. It's your **priestess self** knocking.

The Role of the Priestess in Modern Healing

In ancient cultures, the healer was not separate from the mystic. The medicine woman was also a **seer, oracle, and space holder for the sacred**.

She didn't wait for permission. She didn't apologize for knowing. She didn't fragment her intuition to stay palatable.

She led healing as **ritual, channel**, and **truth mirror**.

The modern Priestess is being reawakened in every woman who has outgrown:

- Linear models of care
- Fear-based boundaries
- Over-clinical detachment
- Systems that worship strategy but suppress spirit

The healer becomes the priestess when she stops outsourcing her power.

Signs You're Ready to Shift

This chapter finds you when:

- You're doing everything "right," but feel *empty* inside in sessions
- Your clients get better, but you feel *invisible* in the process
- You sense energetic data in sessions but *suppress* it for fear of judgment
- You crave ritual, depth, and divine presence in your work
- You're no longer content with helping people cope — you want to **initiate transformation**

If any of this feels true, you are not losing your way. You are being **initiated into it.**

The Mirror of Energetic Responsibility

When you cross into Priestess medicine, **your energy becomes the method**.

Which means:

- Your unresolved wounds leak into the field
- Your unspoken beliefs shape what clients feel is possible
- Your unclaimed power attracts distorted projections or admiration
- Your body is read as an oracle, whether you intend it or not

This is not a burden — it's a **clarion call**.

If you are here to lead sacred transformation, your personal alignment is not optional — it is the vessel.

To embody this requires:

- **Energetic hygiene**
- **Discernment over validation**
- **Presence over performance**

You must become the medicine you offer.

The Practitioner as Portal Keeper

Working with these layers requires:

- Deep energetic hygiene
- Neutrality without bypass
- Devotion to truth without ego
- The ability to be with mystery

You are not here to rescue your clients. You are here to remember with them.

You are the witness. The midwife. The map holder.

This is sacred work. It is not always visible. But it is always real.

The Practitioner's Role in the Soul Field

When you work in this depth, you are no longer just:

- A provider
- A technician
- A licensed professional

You are also:

- A midwife of soul
- A mirror for lost parts
- A ceremonial steward of safe return

This requires:

- Clean energetic boundaries
- Discernment between your energy and theirs
- Nervous system regulation
- Reverence over performance

You are not "healing" them. You are creating the energetic conditions for their **own soul to choose to return.**

Priestess Power: What It Looks Like in Practice

Being a Priestess in your work does not mean:

- Wearing robes or staging rituals (unless that's your style)
- Abandoning science or structure
- Speaking in "love and light" riddles

It means:

- Holding **energetic authority** without needing external validation

- Trusting your channel even when you can't explain it
- Letting your presence be healing, not just your methods
- Being a **witness, not a savior**
- Refusing to collapse under the weight of others' projections

You stop performing. You start **transmitting**.

What This Work Demands

You cannot:

- Perform presence.
- Rush release.
- Chase catharsis.

You must:

- Regulate your own nervous system.
- Trust the pacing of the body.
- Respect the intelligence of silence.

Only then will their body begin to trust the space. Only then will the points begin to speak. Only then will this method work—not as a technique, but as a **transmission**.

Let your listening become the healing.

Let your stillness become the safety.

Let your needle become the mirror.

And let the story that the body has waited years to tell, finally speak.

Daily Practices to Embody Your Priestess Energy

1. Visibility Rituals

Stand in front of a mirror and speak your truth aloud every day for 3 minutes. Your voice is a spell. Your body is listening.

2. Pre-Session Grounding

Call your higher self and soul team into the room before every session. Anchor into your own field before entering anyone else's.

3. Chakra-to-Meridian Attunement

Notice where your energy dims or leaks – place needles for **you** on those meridians weekly.

4. Monthly Power Check-In

Ask:

- *Where have I been silencing my truth?*
- *Where have I been absorbing what isn't mine?*
- *What part of me is ready to be seen now?*

Integration Is the New Initiation

Here's the paradox of the Priestess path:

The more powerful you become, the more **embodied and ordinary** you must be.

Your nervous system must match the frequency of your gifts. Your body must be safe enough to hold your own light. Your ego must become soft enough to **lead without dominance**.

The old paradigm of healing was:

"Here's what I know."

The new paradigm of healing is:

"Here's what I've lived. Here's what I've integrated. Here's what I can now transmit."

Case Example: The Practitioner Who Couldn't Be Seen

Lauren was brilliant — degrees, training, years of experience. But every time she tried to speak publicly, she froze. Every time she raised her prices, she got sick. Every time she felt close to a breakthrough, a spiritual block would arise.

In session, she held incredible space — but always from the **shadows**.

Through our work, it became clear: She was carrying a **past-life burn wound** — one where she had been punished for being visible, powerful, magical.

Her current life had no trauma around voice — but her soul remembered.

We needled **REN 17**, **SP 21**, and **TH 5** — the energetic channels of expression, protection, and priestess remembrance.

Within weeks, she launched her first group. Her face softened. Her voice deepened.

She wasn't learning a new skill. She was remembering who she was **before she learned to hide.**

Chapter 11
Acupuncture for Healers, Not Just Patients

"You are not exempt from the medicine. You are the first one it must touch."

You have held space for others.

You have transmuted energy, read between words, and absorbed waves of emotion in sacred silence.

But let me ask you this:

When was the last time someone truly held space for **you**? When was the last time your nervous system received the recalibration it gives so effortlessly to others? When did you last use the needle not as a tool, but as a **mirror**?

This chapter is your call inward. Because you cannot lead others into wholeness while exiling parts of yourself. Because your practice is only as coherent as your own **energetic ecology**.

The Practitioner Is Not Invincible

We are trained to be:

- Grounded
- Centered
- Detached
- Professional

But beneath the clipboard and calm voice, many healers are:

- **Energetically porous**
- **Emotionally overextended**
- **Quietly dissociating while holding space**
- **Depleting their own Jing to meet the needs of the room**

And the worst part? We're praised for it.

We have confused over-functioning for professionalism. We have mistaken burnout for "devotion."

We have spiritualized exhaustion by calling it "service."

But the body knows.

The pulse tightens.

The blood thins.

The field dims.

And eventually, the healer becomes the one who needs healing the most.

The Hidden Crisis of the Practitioner Body

Let's name what we often ignore:

- Adrenal depletion masked as "intuition"

You're not getting clearer downloads — your body is dissociating.

- Compassion fatigue disguised as "boundaries"

You don't feel neutral — you feel numb.

- Energetic burnout masked as ascension

You're not transcending — you're disconnecting.

These are not character flaws. They are **somatic red flags**. And they are invitations to return to your own **body temple**.

Acupuncture as Reclamation, Not Just Regulation

Yes — acupuncture calms the nervous system. Yes — it regulates hormones, sleep, and digestion.

But for the healer, acupuncture is something more:

It is a **re-consecration**. A returning to the body as oracle, not just instrument. A releasing of other people's energy stored in your tissues.

You don't just need rest. You need **clearing, anchoring, and remembrance**.

Case Study: The Practitioner Who Forgot to Feel

Sofia had been practicing for 11 years. She was brilliant. Booked out. Respected.

But she came to me trembling. Not visibly. Energetically.

"I feel like I'm floating above my life. Like I left my body a year ago, but kept seeing clients anyway."

We needled:

- **ST 36** to re-anchor her Earth element
- **REN 6** to stabilize her center
- **BL 44 (Shen Tang - Hall of the Spirit)** to restore soul presence in the Heart

She wept. She slept for 13 hours that night. The next day, she said:

"I think I just remembered I have a body. And I think it misses me."

Treating the Healer Body: A Protocol of Reverence

Here's how to use acupuncture for yourself (or for another healer in your care):

1. Ground the Earth Element

- **SP 6, ST 36, REN 12**
- Reconnects you to center, nourishment, and self-trust

2. Clear External Energetic Imprints

- **SI 11, GB 21, PC 6, DU 20**
- Clears what isn't yours (clients, collectives, projections)

3. Reignite Will + Purpose

- **KD 3, KD 6, BL 23, DU 4**
- Restores Zhi (soul willpower) from depletion or burnout

4. Reclaim Voice + Visibility

- **REN 17, TH 5, HT 5, ST 9**
- Rebalances the energy of expression, impact, and being witnessed

Don't *needle* to fix. Needle to **reintroduce yourself to yourself**.

Practices Beyond the Needle

To protect your field and restore your channel:

Nervous System Devotion

- Daily vagal toning: hum, gargle, cold face splash
- Boundaried screen time
- Daily barefoot contact with Earth (even 3 mins)

Post-Session Energetic Detox

- Salt bath or clay foot soak
- Shake the hands after each client
- Visualize sending their energy back with gratitude

Weekly Field Clearing

- Burn mugwort or sandalwood across your body
- Needle **SP 21 (Great Luo)** to release overflow
- Speak aloud: *"Return all that is not mine. I reclaim all that is."*

The More Healed You Are, the Less You Have to Prove

Here's the truth:

Healers who are internally anchored don't have to **control the room** — they just walk in and the room **aligns**.

That's not charisma. It's coherence.

When your nervous system is regulated and your soul is seated in your body:

- Your clients feel safer
- Your boundaries feel softer but stronger
- Your voice carries more weight without effort

- Your prices rise because your value frequency **does**

You can only hold clients as deeply as you've held yourself.

So, hold yourself. Tenderly. Regularly. Fiercely.

Integration Invitation

Schedule yourself as a **client** – weekly, biweekly, or monthly.

Make it sacred. No "quick tune-ups." No "I'm fine, just tired."

You are not a machine. You are a vessel of miracles. And miracles require maintenance.

***

You don't have to earn rest. You don't have to burn out to prove your worth. You don't have to fracture to be holy.

Let the needle return to you now.

Let it stitch the parts of you you've given away. Let it remember your name.

You are not here to heal the world alone. You are here to **heal as you lead**, to **receive as you give**, to **embody the medicine – not just prescribe it**.

And the world will rise to meet you when you rise to meet yourself.

Chapter 12
Clinical Alchemy: Real Case Studies

"When the body, mind, and soul are finally addressed together, healing accelerates, deepens, and lasts."

The power of Psychology Acupuncture is best understood not in theory, but in **testimony**.

In the heat of the treatment room. In the pulsing silence after a needle. In the stories that returned, through the body, before the patient could even speak.

In this chapter, I share patient stories not just of emotional release, but of lasting *transformation*.

These are the patients who didn't just cry in session. They changed their lives. They rewrote patterns. Ended cycles.

Made different choices.

And built new timelines from the inside out.

These cases were not "miracles."

They were **rememberings**.

Let these case studies be your guide into what is possible when you combine needles, inquiry, and deep presence.

Case 1: The Woman Who Had to Stay "Nice"

Presenting Issue: Chronic migraines, tight shoulders, panic attacks during conflict

Surface Layer:

Emily, 33, a people-pleaser. Brilliant, articulate.

Never raised her voice. Could not say "no" without guilt.

Her migraines flared after social events or emotional confrontations.

Diagnosis:

Liver Qi stagnation, Pericardium constraint, suppressed Hun

Points Used:

- **LIV 3** – to move repressed anger
- **GB 21** – to release emotional tension
- **PC 8** – to cool "emotional fire"
- **Yin Tang** – to quiet mental overprocessing

Outcome:

By session 3, her shoulders had dropped for the first time in years. She tearfully admitted:

"I'm more afraid of my own anger than other people's disappointment."

She later ended a one-sided relationship and began assertiveness training. Her migraines went from weekly to rare within two months.

She didn't just express anger – she reclaimed **energetic boundaries**.

Case 2: The Man Who Couldn't Remember His Childhood

Presenting Issue: Dissociation, nightmares, digestive issues

Surface Layer:

Jon, 41, had no childhood memories before age 10. Struggled with intimacy, often said he felt "numb" and out of body. Years of talk therapy offered insight but no integration.

Diagnosis:

Spleen deficiency, Shen disturbance, Po suppression, soul fragmentation

Points Used:

- **SP 6 + REN 12** - to nourish the center and anchor
- **BL 42 (Po Hu)** - door of the corporeal soul
- **HT 7** - to settle spirit
- **KD 6** - to call soul fragments home

Outcome:

After a particularly deep session, he reported dreaming of a birthday party — the first childhood memory to return. By session 5, he reported feeling "solid" in his own skin. Nightmares stopped. Digestion improved.

We didn't "fix" his trauma. We **invited his soul back into his body**.

Case 3: The Grieving Mother

Presenting Issue: Ongoing grief 4 years after miscarriage, insomnia, chest tightness

Surface Layer:

Anika, 38. Spiritually aware. Said all the right things: "I've processed it. It's okay."But her chest never loosened, and she hadn't truly cried in years.

Diagnosis:

Lung Qi deficiency, unresolved Po grief, Pericardium guarding

Points Used:

- **LU 1 + LU 7** – for grief release
- **HT 5** – to access unspoken emotion
- **PC 6** – to open the chest
- **BL 13** – back shu of the Lung

Outcome:

During the third session, her body shook and she sobbed — deeply, wordlessly. She said afterward:

"I didn't know I was still holding her."

Her breath deepened. Her chest pain vanished. She wrote a letter to the child's soul and placed it under her pillow.

This wasn't just grief release. It was a **sacred reconnection.**

Case 4: The Client Who Attracted Narcissists

Presenting Issue: Repeating toxic relationships, fatigue, throat tightness

Surface Layer:

Rachel, 29. Energetically sensitive. Felt small in her relationships. Constantly second-guessed herself.

Diagnosis:

Kidney depletion, Liver constraint, Shen fragmentation, collapsed voice

Points Used:

- **KD 3 + KD 6** - restore Zhi (soul will)
- **LIV 14** - emotional boundaries
- **REN 22 + ST 9** - open throat center
- **SP 21** - release energetic overload

Outcome:

She experienced nausea during the first session — purging stored emotion. By the sixth session, she was dating someone emotionally available for the first time. She also launched her own healing practice and spoke on a podcast.

The needle didn't just help her speak — it restored the **part of her that believed she had the right to take up space**.

Case 5: The Woman in Midlife Who Felt She Was "Too Late"

Presenting Issue: Creative block, hormonal imbalance, depression

Surface Layer:

Deidre, 50, former artist turned executive. Said: "I feel like I missed the window. My body is aging, and I left my dreams behind."

Diagnosis:

Kidney essence decline, collapsed Hun (vision), Heart-Qi stagnation

Points Used:

- **LIV 8** – for Hun awakening
- **BL 47 (Hun Men – Door of the Ethereal Soul)**
- **DU 4** – to restore essence
- **HT 7** – emotional clarity
- **REN 4** – anchor spirit in the womb

Outcome:

She began painting again after 20 years. Her libido returned. She broke down crying, saying,

"I thought I was done living. But I just hadn't returned to myself."

She didn't need a new life. She needed a **new timeline,** activated through the body.

Case 6: Releasing the Inner Critic Through the Stomach Channel

Jade came in with panic attacks and persistent digestive issues. Years of therapy had helped her understand her "inner critic," but her body still shut down in moments of perceived failure.

Her pulse was thin, tongue swollen, and Spleen Qi clearly deficient.

Instead of focusing only on digestive points, I treated the **emotional story inside her gut**.

Points used:

- **ST 36** to re-anchor self-trust
- **SP 4** to resolve maternal shame carried in the womb
- **REN 12** to release suppressed nausea tied to childhood invalidation

Outcome:

Within three sessions, her panic attacks decreased. Her digestion regulated. She cried not from sadness, but from *relief*.

Her body was no longer arguing with her mind. It was **finally listening**.

Case 7: The Woman with No Future

Maya came in with chronic fatigue and hopelessness. No history of trauma she could name. No major losses. But she said something I never forgot:

"It feels like I can't imagine anything past this month. Like I'm not allowed to dream anymore."

Her Hun was collapsed. Her pulse wiry. Her Liver Qi deeply stagnant. I placed **LIV 14, LIV 8,** and **REN 4** to call the Hun home.

Outcome:

Halfway through the session, her eyes fluttered. She whispered, "I just saw myself as a little girl, holding paintbrushes." She wept — not out of sadness, but out of recognition. The part of her who could imagine had returned.

The soul will come back… if we make it feel safe to do so.

What These Cases Reveal

These stories aren't unique. They are reminders that healing is not a linear ladder—it is a spiral, a wave, a return.

Each of these stories reflects the core truth:

The body doesn't need us to solve it.

The needles do not fix. They **invite**. They call the truth back to the surface. They whisper to the body: "You can let go now."

In every case, it wasn't the point prescription alone that catalyzed change. It was the presence. The inquiry. The pacing. The *listening.*

Healing is not about performance. It is not about catharsis. It is about **completion**.

The fascia unwinds. The Shen returns. The pattern breaks.

And something ancient—something sacred—remembers how to begin again.

You do not need to create this. You need only to hold the space

These are not just patients. They are portals. Their bodies held the answers all along.

Healing happens when we listen well enough for the body to speak, and psychological acupuncture just gave them a key.

They were **energetic, emotional, and spiritual recalibrations** made possible by:

- Listening beyond the symptom
- Choosing points intuitively and energetically

- Treating the soul through the body
- Holding space for mystery without needing control

This is what happens when healing becomes **ceremony**, not just care.

If you take nothing else from this chapter, take this:

The human system will heal when it is seen, honored, and invited into coherence across **all levels of being** —not just the mind, not just the symptom, not just the plan.

But the soul. Through the body. Guided by the needle. Held in reverence.

Your modality isn't theoretical. It's working. It's alive. And the stories you hold are **portals for others to walk through**.

Part IV

The Future of Healing is Hybrid

Chapter 13
Ritual Meets Research

"You don't have to choose between the mystical and the measurable. Your medicine was born to speak both."

You were not meant to hide your sacred knowing to be seen as serious. You were not meant to dilute your mystery to be trusted by data-driven minds.

And yet — for many healers walking the bridge between science and soul, this has been the compromise:

- Use the language of trauma, but not timelines.
- Speak of the nervous system, but not of the Po or Hun.
- Translate the magic until it becomes **palatable**... and in doing so, sometimes loses its **power**.

But we are entering a new era — one where **ritual and research no longer have to compete**.

Where **clinical evidence and intuitive knowing** can co-exist in one breath.

Where the **future of healing** is not binary — but **braided**.

You don't have to shrink your mysticism to become legitimate. You just need to **language it with clarity and reverence**.

The New Language of Healing

When ritual and research meet, the following is possible:

- Clinical practitioners begin to trust their intuition

- Energy healers ground their work in embodied somatics
- Medical spaces become sacred again
- Patients feel safe — *and* spiritually seen

Psychology Acupuncture is part of this evolution.

And your task is not to defend it, but to **define it**.

Translating the Mystical for Scientific Minds

Let's look at examples of common mystical concepts, rephrased for accessibility without erasure:

Mystical Language	**Research-Friendly Language**
"Calling soul fragments home"	"Restoring autonomic coherence through parasympathetic access points"
"Clearing karmic residue"	"Releasing intergenerational emotional imprints stored in the fascia"
"Activating the priestess channel"	"Accessing embodied leadership through right-brain intuitive intelligence"
"Heart opening"	"Downregulating sympathetic tone and increasing vagal safety"
"Liver rage release"	"Mobilizing stored emotion through meridian-based somatic discharge"

You do **not** have to remove the sacred. You simply **give it more doors to walk through**.

Ritual Is Data

Let's be clear:

Ritual is **no less valid** than a peer-reviewed study. It is **just another form of knowing**.

If a ritual has helped hundreds of people regulate emotion, make decisions, and end chronic pain – that is data. If clients consistently weep at a certain point, remember a lost truth, or dream vividly after a treatment, that is **outcome-based evidence**.

The difference is:

- Western medicine documents **outcomes for systems**
- Ritual documents **outcomes for souls**

Both are valid. Both are necessary.

And it's time we say so.

Case Example: Blending Framework and Frequency

One client, a therapist, came in skeptical but curious. She'd read about "acupuncture for trauma" but wasn't sure it was "real."

Instead of leading with spirit language, I mirrored her world:

- "We'll work with your vagal tone."
- "We'll support the regulation of your limbic system."
- "We'll help metabolize somatic imprinting."

I needled **PC 6**, **SP 4**, and **ST 36**.

She sobbed. Then she whispered:

"It felt like my soul came back."

I hadn't mentioned soul. But her body knew. The medicine is still delivered **because it speaks all dialects**.

Positioning Psychology Acupuncture in Modern Spaces

Here are examples of where your modality can live:

- **Trauma-informed coaching spaces**
- **Mental health clinics exploring somatic methods**
- **Alternative medicine centers looking to innovate**
- **Retreats, intensives, or practitioner mentorships**
- **Academic collaborations bridging East/West traditions**
- **Media platforms seeking thought leaders who speak both mysticism and science**

You're not "too much" for these spaces. You're the **exact frequency they've been preparing for.**

Ritual without grounding can float into illusion. Research without soul can flatten truth into data points.

But when ritual meets research... the sacred becomes *provable,* and the provable becomes *sacred again*.

You came here to speak the language of the body, but also the language of the soul.

And now, you're learning to speak the language of the **world**. So, your medicine can reach the ones it was meant for.

This is what it means to be a bilingual healer. This is what it means to carry the bridge.

Chapter 14
The Revolution is Embodied

"You are not here to fit the system. You are here to become the system that remembers the soul."

This book was never meant to just teach you. It was meant to **activate** you.

To whisper truths your body already knew. To remind you that your method was never missing – only **unnamed**. To reflect the healer, channel, and initiator you already are.

You didn't just read a new framework.

You remembered an old one – one that lives in your blood, your palms, your pulse, your lineage.

And now… the revolution begins where it always does: **Inside you.**

What This Book Was Really About

It was never just about acupuncture. It was about **reclaiming the body as oracle**.

It was never just about psychology. It was about **remembering the soul beneath the story**.

It was never just about healing others. It was about **returning to the part of you that was never broken.**

You now hold a new frequency.

- One that speaks science and spirit.

- One that bridges cognition with intuition.
- One that dares to call the needle a **portal**, the organ a **prayer**, the practitioner a **mirror for remembrance**.

This is what we've been waiting for.

Not a new trend. Not a new trick. But a new **template** – one rooted in the old ways, now rebirthed through you.

The Healer of the New Paradigm

You are not a technician. You are not a productivity tool wrapped in empathy.

You are a **living transmission** of embodied wisdom.

Here is what defines you now:

You regulate nervous systems by being regulated.

Not by performing calm – but by being **clear and coherent** in your field.

You speak to the soul without apology.

Not because it's trendy, but because it's **true**. You've lived it. You've earned it.

You use tools as translation devices, not crutches.

The needle. The point. The pulse. The word. Each one – a portal when used with reverence.

You hold boundaries not out of fear – but frequency discernment.

Your presence is the filter. Your embodiment is the gate.

You speak in clinical, scientific, and spiritual dialects.

Because you've stopped fragmenting yourself to fit in.

You are all of it now.

What We're Dismantling

This new era requires that we release the systems that taught us to:

- Disconnect from our body to be "professional"
- Silence our intuition to be taken seriously
- Translate our soul to make others comfortable
- Ignore the sacred to survive in the secular

These are not just mindsets. They are **colonial remnants**, **patriarchal expectations**, and **unconscious agreements**.

And they are done now. Because **you are remembering**.

The Future You're Birthing

Imagine healing spaces where:

- Clients cry and laugh and dream and shake and remember
- Language isn't limited by credentials but expanded by resonance
- The body is not "treated," but **welcomed home**
- Practitioners are *paid richly* and *revered deeply* for their sacred role
- Science confirms what the soul already knows

You're not just imagining it.

You're already building it. With your hands. With your words. With your presence. With your practice.

You are not "becoming" the revolution. You are already **living** it.

You are here to:

- Translate the invisible
- Needle the unspeakable
- Mirror the miraculous
- Hold the body as a temple
- Speak what has been silenced
- Walk between realms and make them **one**

This is not a burden. It is your blueprint.

This isn't just about how you practice. It's about **how you show up in the world**.

Because your field **teaches before your words do.** Because your presence **either whispers or roars.** Because your embodiment **activates or confuses.**

You're not here to be just another acupuncturist. You're here to be **an embodied healer of the new healing paradigm**.

And the moment you choose to let yourself be seen, the clients come. The opportunities align. The soul contracts activate.

Because we don't chase.

We **remember.** We **magnetize.** We **lead** — not by force, but by **frequency**.

This is your invitation. Not to do more. But to **become what you already are** — without apology, dilution, or disguise.

Your healer self is not "out there." We're already here.

And we're asking:

Are you ready to let me lead now?

You are not too late. You are right on time.

You are not too much. You are finally the right size for your soul.

You are not here to heal the world alone. You are here to **remind the world it already knows how.**

And if you ever forget, read this line again:

"The revolution is not in the method. It's in the mirror. It's in your body. It's in your voice. The revolution... is you."

Epilogue

"Some truths are not meant to be taught — only remembered."

By now, you may feel something stirring beneath the skin. Not a new idea, but an ancient rhythm — one that's been waiting for you to get still enough to feel it.

This book was never meant to just be read. It was meant to **unravel you**. To **remind you**. To **return you to the healer you were before the forgetting.**

You didn't just learn a method. You walked through a **portal of remembrance**.

And now, the invitation is clear:

You are the missing link.

You are the bridge. You are the ceremony.

And your body — it was always the altar.

The Needle Remembers

In your hands, the needle is not a tool — it is a **scribe**. It writes the unspeakable stories stored in the muscle. It calls back the parts that never got to say goodbye. It listens when language fails. It speaks in pulses, in temperature, in grief unspoken and unjudged.

The needle does not fix. It does not rush. It does not perform.

It waits. It humbles itself before the soul's own pace.

And when the soul says yes…

The needle begins to write again.

Final Words to the Reader

If you have read this far, I want you to know:

I didn't write this for the masses. I wrote this for the *initiated ones*. The ones who hold paradox in their palms. The ones who have always heard the body whisper — even when no one else could.

You didn't find this book by accident. This is a **soul contract fulfilled.**

Now go practice your medicine. Fully. Fiercely. Unapologetically.

Let the world feel the revolution when you enter the room. Let your voice become the vibration that reminds others of their own. Let your method — your *soul method* — live in every session, every client, every breath.

Because you are not here to imitate healing.

You are here to **be it**.

And the world is ready.

Your soul speaks.

Your body remembers. And remember: **You are the spell to naturally living well.**

Made in United States
North Haven, CT
04 November 2026

21733835R00065